NCLEX: Gastrointestinal Disorders

Easily Dominate the Test with 105 Practice Questions & Rationales to Help You Become a Nurse!

Chase Hassen
Nurse Superhero
© 2016

Disclaimer:

Although the author and publisher have made every effort to ensure that the information in this book was correct at press time, the author and publisher do not assume and hereby disclaim any liability to any party for any loss, damage, or disruption caused by errors or omissions, whether such errors or omissions result from negligence, accident, or any other cause.

This book is not intended as a substitute for the medical advice of physicians. The reader should regularly consult a physician in matters relating to his/her health and particularly with respect to any symptoms that may require diagnosis or medical attention.

All rights reserved. No part of this publication may be reproduced, distributed, or transmitted in any form or by any means, including photocopying, recording, or other electronic or mechanical methods, without the prior written permission of the publisher, except in the case of brief quotations embodied in critical reviews and certain other noncommercial uses permitted by copyright law.

NCLEX®, NCLEX®-RN, and NCLEX®-PN are registered trademarks of the National Council of State Boards of Nursing, Inc. They hold no affiliation with this product.

© **Copyright 2016 by Chase Hassen & Nurse Superhero.
All rights reserved.**

TABLE OF CONTENTS

Chapter 1 : NCLEX-RN : Gastrointestinal Questions, Answers, and Rationales 1

Conclusion 53

First, I want to give you this FREE gift…

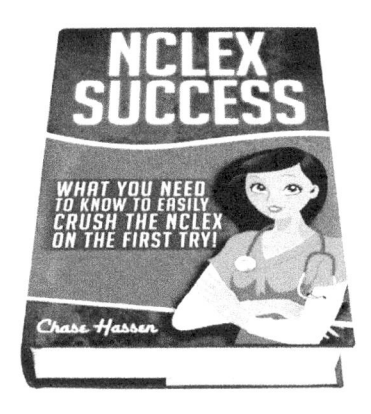

Just to say thanks for downloading my book, I wanted to give you another resource to help you absolutely crush the NCLEX Exam.

For a limited time, you can download this book for FREE.
http://bit.ly/1VvK2e7 .

CHAPTER 1 :
NCLEX-RN : GASTROINTESTINAL QUESTIONS, ANSWERS, AND RATIONALES

The following are 105 questions that will help you study for the NCLEX evaluation. All of the questions are based on suggestions you may see on the test. Compare your answers with the correct answers to see where you may need to study further. Good luck!

1. The client has right upper quadrant pain, nausea and fever. What is the most likely diagnosis?
   a. Appendicitis
   b. Irritable bowel syndrome
   c. Acute cholecystitis
   d. Acute gastritis

Answer: c. The gallbladder is located in the right upper quadrant and when it becomes inflamed, you get right upper quadrant abdominal pain, nausea, fever, and clay colored stools.

2. The client has severe upper abdominal pain, nausea and vomiting, and an elevated amylase and lipase. What is the likely diagnosis?
   a. Acute cholecystitis
   b. Chronic gastritis
   c. Liver cirrhosis
   d. Acute pancreatitis

Answer: d. Abdominal pain, nausea and vomiting, along with an elevated amylase and lipase usually means the client has acute pancreatitis.

3. The client is to have an oral cholecystogram. The purpose of the oral cholecystogram is what?
   a. To evaluate levels of pancreatic secretions.
   b. To assess the ability of the gallbladder to concentrate, contract, and empty.
   c. To evaluate duodenal digestion.
   d. To look for acute cholecystitis

Answer: b. The purpose of the oral cholecystogram is to evaluate the gallbladder and its ability to concentrate, contract, and empty.

4. The client is to have an oral cholecystogram. What pre-procedure nursing tasks should be done? Check all that apply.
   a. Check for allergy to seafood or iodine.
   b. Order a high fat diet for the client.
   c. Check a bilirubin level.
   d. Give one Telepaque tablet 2 hours after dinner.
   e. Give a high fat diet just before procedure.
   f. Tell the radiologist about vomiting or diarrhea after dye ingestion.

Answer: a. c. f. The day before the procedure, the nurse checks for allergy to seafood or iodine, orders a low fat diet for the client, checks a bilirubin because the test can't be done if the bilirubin is above 2.0, gives 6 Telepaque tablets two hours after the dinner. The radiologist should be informed of vomiting or diarrhea after dye ingestion. The patient is to be NPO after receiving the dye.

5. The client is scheduled for a cholangiogram. What is the purpose of the test?
   a. To evaluate the excretion of the gallbladder.
   b. To evaluate excretion of bile from the common bile duct.
   c. To assess the patency of the hepatic and common bile duct.
   d. To evaluate pancreatic secretions.

Answer: c. The purpose of the cholangiogram is to evaluate the patency of the hepatic and common bile duct.

6. The client is scheduled for a cholangiogram. What are some pre-procedure nursing tasks? Select all that apply.
   1. Light meal the morning of the test.
   2. Assess for allergy to seafood or iodine.
   3. Oral radiographic dye given the morning of the test.
   4. Assess bilirubin level
   5. NPO after midnight
   6. Drink 6 glasses of water before test.

Answer: b. d. e. The day before the test, assess for allergy to seafood or iodine and get a bilirubin test. If the bilirubin is greater than 3.5 mg/dL, you can't do the test. The patient is to be NPO after midnight and the radiographic dye is given intravenously.

7. The client is having an upper GI series. Nursing tasks to be done before the procedure include:
   a. Fat free meal before the procedure
   b. Assess allergy to seafood or iodine
   c. NPO for 8-12 hours before the procedure
   d. Laxative given before procedure

Answer: c. The client should be NPO for 8-12 hours before the procedure. No smoking. The contrast is barium so there is no allergy potential. The laxative is given after the procedure is done.

8. After an upper GI series, the nursing tasks to be done include the following:
   a. Limit fluid intake
   b. Watch for allergies to contrast dye
   c. NPO for 12 hours post procedure
   d. Provide a laxative to get rid of the barium

Answer: d. After the procedure, encourage 6-8 glasses of water per day, eating can be normal and a laxative should be provided to get rid of the barium. Stools may be white for up to 72 hours.

9. The client is scheduled for a Barium Enema. Nursing tasks before the procedure include:
   a. Fluid restriction the day before the procedure
   b. Clear liquid for lunch and dinner the day before procedure
   c. 8 ounces of fluid every hour for 8-10 hours
   d. Assess for allergies to shellfish or iodine
   e. 10 ounces of magnesium citrate in mid to late afternoon before the procedure
   f. Biscodyl tablets given the day before the procedure

Answer: b. c. e. f. The client should have a clear liquid lunch and dinner before procedure, and they must drink an 8 oz. glass of fluid every hour for 8-10 hours. 10 oz. of magnesium citrate is given in the mid to late afternoon before the procedure. Biscodyl tablets given the day before the procedure.

10. The client is scheduled for an ERCP. What nursing tasks are done before the procedure? Select all that apply.
    a. NPO after midnight
    b. Withhold sedatives at the time of the procedure
    c. Tell the client that breathing will not be compromised by the endoscope
    d. Nonfat diet the day of the test
    e. Tell the client to lie very still so ducts can be seen
    f. Remove the client's dentures before the test.

Answer: a. c. e. f. The patient should be NPO after midnight and should have a sedative for the test. The client should know that breathing will not be compromised by the endoscope. The client should lie very still so the ducts can be seen. Dentures should be removed.

11. Following an ERCP, the nursing tasks should be as follows. Select all that apply.
    a. May eat immediately after procedure.
    b. Monitor for ERCP-related pancreatitis.
    c. Provide laxatives after the procedure.
    d. Maintain bedrest with side rails up after the procedure
    e. Drink 8 glasses of water after procedure
    f. Provide throat lozenges after procedure.

Answer: b. d. f. After the procedure, the patient should be NPO until anesthetic wears off. Monitor for ERCP-related pancreatitis. Bedrest with side rails up until sedative wears off. Provide throat lozenges or warm saltwater gargles for relief of sore throat.

12. The purpose of a colonoscopy is what?
    a. To visualize the sigmoid colon
    b. To visualize the small intestines
    c. To visualize the duodenum
    d. To visualize the large bowel

Answer: d. The purpose of a colonoscopy is to visualize the entire large bowel from the rectum to the cecum.

13. Prior to a colonoscopy, the nursing tasks include the following. Select all that apply.
    a. Give a gallon of GoLYTELY the evening before the procedure.
    b. NPO 12 hours before procedure.
    c. Give Biscodyl Tablets the night before.
    d. Assess for allergy to contrast dye.
    e. Clear liquid diet up until 8 hours before procedure.
    f. Low fat meal the morning of the procedure.

Answer: a. c. e. The nurse gives a gallon of GoLYTELY the evening before the procedure and allows for a clear liquid diet up until 8 hours pre-procedure and then NPO. Biscodyl is given the night before the procedure. The test does not involve contrast dye.

14. An upper GI Endoscopy visualizes what part of the GI tract? Select all that apply.
    a. *Esophagus*
    b. *Stomach*
    c. *Duodenum*
    d. *Small bowel*
    e. *Appendix*
    f. *Large bowel*

Answer: a. b. c. The upper GI endoscopy can visualize the esophagus, stomach and sometimes the duodenum.

15. The client is having a liver biopsy. What can be done to assure the biopsy can be taken?
    a. *Have the client exhale and hold the exhalation to allow the liver to descend*
    b. *Place the client on the right side*
    c. *Have the client cough to bring the liver down*
    d. *Place the patient on the left side*

Answer: a. To bring the liver down, the client must exhale and hold the exhalation so the liver can be exposed.

16. The client is scheduled for a gastric analysis. What is the purpose of this test?
    a. To assess the amount of intrinsic factor in the stomach.
    b. To assess the basal and maximal acid output
    c. To assess the concentration of pepsinogen in the stomach
    d. To biopsy the stomach lining

Answer: b. A gastric analysis assesses the basal and maximal acid output in the stomach.

17. What is the order of the steps in the gastric analysis procedure?
    a. Take four samples of the maximum output.
    b. Insert a nasogastric tube.
    c. Give subcutaneous histamine.
    d. Take four samples of the basal acid output.

Answer: b. d. c. a. First you insert the nasogastric tube and then you take four samples of the basal acid output. Then give subcutaneous histamine and take four samples of the maximum acid output.

18. What best describes a gastric emptying study?
    a. It is a radionuclide study that scans the stomach emptying
    b. It involves a small camera at the end of a flexible tube.
    c. It involves drinking barium and watching the stomach empty.
    d. It involves a contrast medium taken orally to assess stomach emptying.

Answer: a. It is a radionuclide study in which the individual takes in a liquid or solid meal laced with Technetium.

19. After a colonoscopy, what are some nursing tasks?
    a. Ambulate after the procedure
    b. Monitor for signs of colon perforation
    c. Offer food when no evidence of colon perforation
    d. Offer laxatives
    e. Provide fluids to rehydrate
    f. Offer anti-emetics

Answer: b. c. e. After a colonoscopy, the client needs bedrest until sedative wears off. Monitor for signs of colon perforation and if none, offer food. Provide fluids to rehydrate the client. Laxatives and anti-emetics are not necessary.

20. The client is having a proctosigmoidoscopy. What is the preparation for the test?
    a. Drink a gallon of GoLYTELY the night before the test.
    b. Administer an enema the evening before the procedure.
    c. Clear liquids for 24 hours prior to the procedure.
    d. Biscodyl tablets the night before the procedure.

Answer: b. To prepare for the proctosigmoidoscopy, the client needs to have an enema the evening before the procedure.

21. The Hemoccult slide test has several steps. Put them in the order they are performed.
    a. Open the front cover of the Hemoccult slide.
    b. Have the client defecate into an appropriate container.
    c. Look for bluish discoloration on the slide.
    d. Smear stool on the front of the Hemoccult slide.
    e. Open the back of the Hemoccult slide and apply two drops of developer

Answer: b. a. d. e. c. First the client defecates into an appropriate container. Then you open the front cover of the Hemoccult slide and smear stool on it. Then you open the back of the slide and apply two drops of developer, looking for bluish discoloration on the slide.

22. The client is scheduled for a urea breath test. What does the test detect?
    a. The presence of Helicobacter pylori
    b. The amount of acid in the stomach
    c. Blood in the GI tract
    d. The presence of stomach ulcers

Answer: a. The test uses radioactive urea to detect the presence of Helicobacter pylori.

23. How is a fecal fat test performed?
    a. A sample of stool is evaluated for fat content.
    b. A smear of stool is placed on a test kit and analyzed for fat content.
    c. Stool is collected over three days and fat content is determined.
    d. Stool from one bowel movement is assessed for fat content.

Answer: c. In a fecal fat test, stool is collected continuously for three days and the fat content is determined.

24. The client is scheduled for a paracentesis. What does the nurse say to educate the client about the procedure?
    a. A sample of liver tissue will be taken.
    b. There is a high risk of bleeding.
    c. A needle is inserted to remove ascitic fluid.
    d. A needle is inserted into the bladder to collect sterile urine.

Answer: c. The paracentesis involves inserting a needle into the abdominal cavity to remove fluid in a client with ascites.

25. The best test for acute pancreatitis is what?
    a. Lipase
    b. Amylase
    c. LDH
    d. SGOT

Answer: a. The lipase level is the best test for acute pancreatitis. It is seen as elevated in acute pancreatitis.

26. The test most likely to be elevated in biliary obstruction is what?
    a. Lipase
    b. SGOT
    c. SGPT
    d. Alkaline Phosphatase

Answer: d. In a situation of biliary obstruction, the alkaline phosphatase is most likely to be elevated.

27. Diagnostic tests for GERD include the following. Select all that apply.
   a. Upper GI endoscopy
   b. Esophagoscopy
   c. Esophageal manometry
   d. Urea breath test
   e. Esophageal acid monitoring
   f. Barium swallow

Answer: b. c. e. f. Tests to evaluate a client with GERD include an esophagoscopy, esophageal manometry, esophageal acid monitoring, and barium swallow.

28. The client needs a nasogastric tube. What steps and in what order are the steps taken to place the tube?
   a. Offer the client small sips of water.
   b. Measure the length of the tube to be inserted.
   c. Have the client hyperextend the neck.
   d. Check the pH of the aspirated contents of the tube.
   e. Have the client tilt the head forward.

Answer: b. c. e. a. d. First measure the length of the tube. Have the client hyperextend the neck until he feels the tube in the back of the throat. Then have him tilt the head forward and sip water to facilitate passage of the tube into the esophagus. Measure the pH of the aspirated contents of the tube.

29. A surgical treatment for GERD includes what procedure?
    a. Partial gastrectomy
    b. Nissen fundoplication
    c. Laparoscopic gastrectomy
    d. Esophageal wrap procedure

Answer: b. This procedure is often done laparoscopically and It involves wrapping the fundus of the stomach around the esophagus to tighten the sphincter.

30. A client has esophagitis. The nurse explains the causes of esophagitis to the client as being some of the following. Select all that apply.
    a. Stomach acid
    b. Chemical irritants
    c. Carbonated beverages
    d. Smoking
    e. Alcohol
    f. Temperature extremes of food and fluids

Answer: b. d. e. f. Causes of esophagitis include chemical irritants, smoking, alcohol, and extremes of temperature in food and fluids.

31. A client has a serious complication of chronic acid entering the esophagus over many years. What is this called?
    a. *Esophagitis*
    b. *Heartburn*
    c. *GERD*
    d. *Barrett's esophagus*

Answer: d. Barrett's esophagus is a serious condition that can lead to esophageal cancer caused by chronic amounts of acid entering the esophagus over many years.

32. The client has a hiatal hernia. How does the nurse describe this to the client?
    a. *A part of the abdominal contents has exited the femoral canal.*
    b. *A part of the stomach has exited through the diaphragm.*
    c. *A part of the abdominal contents has exited the inguinal canal.*
    d. *A part of the abdominal contents has exited through the abdominal wall.*

Answer: b. In a hiatal hernia, a part of the stomach has pushed up through a hole in the diaphragm. If the abdominal contents has exited through the femoral canal, it is called a femoral hernia; if the abdominal contents has exited through the inguinal canal, it is called an inguinal hernia; if part o the abdominal contents has exited through the abdominal wall, it is called a ventral hernia.

33. A client has GERD. What nursing instructions should the nurse give upon discharge?
    a. Raise the foot of the bed 4-6 inches.
    b. Quit smoking
    c. Eat large meals
    d. Lose weight
    e. Quit drinking
    f. Don't eat within 4 hours of retiring

Answer: b. d. e. For the management of GERD, the head of the bed should be raised 4-6 inches, the client should eat small meals, quit smoking, quit drinking, lose weight, and should not eat within 4 hours of retiring.

34. A client has peptic ulcer disease. You explain to the patient that the most common site of a peptic ulcer disease is what?
    a. Esophagus
    b. Stomach
    c. Duodenum
    d. Jejunum

Answer: b. While a peptic ulcer can occur in any of the above places, the stomach is more acidic and more prone to peptic ulcer disease.

35. The client has a chronic peptic ulcer and wants to know the difference between an acute and chronic peptic ulcer. How does the nurse educate the client?
    a. An acute ulcer lasts only a month and a chronic ulcer lasts longer than a month.
    b. An acute ulcer is treated with H2 blockers while a chronic ulcer is treated with proton pump inhibitors.
    c. An acute ulcer does not contain H. pylori and a chronic ulcer does.
    d. An acute ulcer is a superficial erosion, while a chronic ulcer extends through the muscular wall of the stomach.

Answer: d. An acute ulcer is a superficial erosion, while a chronic ulcer extends through the muscular wall of the stomach.

36. The client has a gastric ulcer. What do you tell the client as a part of education about the disorder? Select all that apply.
    a. It is a chronic ulcer of longstanding origin.
    b. It occurs more often in men who are 20-30 years of age.
    c. It is more common in those of a lower socioeconomic class.
    d. It is caused by smoking, drug, and alcohol abuse.
    e. It can be caused by the use of NSAIDS or steroids.
    f. It can be caused by H2 blocker use.

Answer: c. d. e. A gastric ulcer is an acute ulceration occurring more commonly in women who are 50-60 years of age and of a lower socioeconomic status. It is caused by smoking, drug use, alcohol use, NSAID use, steroid use, and those suffering from burns or major surgery. It is not caused by H2 blocker use.

37. A client has a gastric ulcer. What are the clinical manifestations you can expect? Select all that apply.
    a. Lower abdominal pain
    b. Pain or gaseous pressure on an empty stomach
    c. Nausea and vomiting
    d. Weight loss
    e. Pain relieved by NSAIDs
    f. Left upper quadrant pain or back pain

Answering: c. d. f. A gastric ulcer involves left upper quadrant or back pain or a sensation of gaseous pressure that occurs 1-2 hours after eating. It can be associated with weight loss.

38. A nurse is caring for someone who has a gastric ulcer. What are some nursing interventions? Select all that apply.
    a. Place the patient on NPO status.
    b. Provide an NG tube.
    c. Use NSAIDs to manage the pain.
    d. Restrict fluids, especially carbonated beverages.
    e. Give antacids or H2 antagonists.
    f. Withhold antibiotics.

Answer: a. b. e. In caring for someone with an acute gastric ulcer, the nurse places the patient on NPO status, provides an NG tube, gives extra fluids and electrolytes, gives antacids or H2 antagonists and gives antibiotics if H. pylori positive.

39. What is a priority nursing intervention in acute hemorrhagic gastric ulcer clients?
    a. Instruct on proper eating habits
    b. Give fluid and electrolytes
    c. Give blood if low hemoglobin
    d. Give NSAIDs for pain

Answer: c. A priority item for acute hemorrhagic gastric ulcer is to give blood for low hemoglobin. Fluid and electrolytes can be given and the nurse should instruct the client on proper eating habits but these are not priority. NSAIDs are contraindicated in acute hemorrhagic gastric ulcers.

40. A client has atrophic gastritis. What does the nurse say as part of education to the client?
    a. Vitamin B6 supplementation is indicated.
    b. There is a loss of intrinsic factor.
    c. It involves a superficial ulcer of the stomach.
    d. Ibuprofen can be given for pain.

Answer: b. Atrophic gastritis involves a severe loss of the lining of the lung so that intrinsic factor cannot be made. Ibuprofen is contraindicated. B12 injections may be necessary for life.

41. The client has atrophic gastritis. What diagnostic tests can confirm the diagnosis?
    a. Colonoscopy
    b. B12 level
    c. Parietal cell antibody test
    d. Intrinsic factor serum test
    e. Upper GI endoscopy
    f. Esophagoscopy

Answer: c. d. e. To test for atrophic gastritis, you can check a parietal cell antibody test and an intrinsic factor serum test. A B12 level might not indicate a cause for low B12 levels and tests like a colonoscopy and esophagoscopy will not identify atrophic gastritis.

42. Nursing interventions upon discharging a client with atrophic gastritis include the following:
    a. Have close monitoring because of a high incidence of gastric cancer.
    b. Expect some gastric bleeding.
    c. Use NSAIDs for arthritic pain or fever
    d. Take laxatives for constipation.

Answer: a. Clients with atrophic gastritis are at high risk for gastric cancer. Bleeding is uncommon and NSAIDs are contraindicated. People with atrophic gastritis have no greater incidence of constipation.

43. A client is having a massive upper GI bleed. What do you tell the client?
    a. You have a 20 percent chance of death.
    b. Your stools should be clay-colored.
    c. You have lost at least 1500 cc of blood.
    d. The bleeding will stop spontaneously.

Answer: c. A massive upper GI bleed is a bleed greater than 1500 cc. There is a 10 percent chance of mortality. The stools are black in color and it may or may not stop spontaneously.

44. A test used to diagnose an upper GI bleed is what?
    a. Angiography of the abdomen
    b. Colonoscopy
    c. Hemoglobin
    d. O2 saturation

Answer: Tests used for the diagnosis of an upper GI bleed is fiberoptic panendoscopy and an angiogram. A colonoscopy alone will not be diagnostic and a low hemoglobin can be from other sources. The O2 saturation can be low but can be due to other causes.

45. A nursing intervention for someone with a gastric outlet obstruction includes this:
    a. Give oral Tylenol for discomfort.
    b. Feed small meals.
    c. Provide an NG tube to continuous suction.
    d. Feed only fluids.
    e. e.

Answer: c. The client with a gastric outlet obstruction should be NPO with nasogastric suction to continuous suction. No oral medication, food, or fluids can be given until the gastric contents come back at less than 200 cc after clamping for 8-12 hours.

46. What are the criteria for surgical intervention for peptic ulcers? Select all that apply.
    a. Drug-induced ulcer
    b. The presence of a duodenal ulcer
    c. The presence of a malignancy
    d. Gastrointestinal bleeding
    e. Control with proton pump inhibitors
    f. Repeated recurrences of ulcer

Answer: a. c. f. The criteria for a surgical management of peptic ulcer include failure of the ulcer to heal, recurrences of ulcer, the presence of a malignancy, or the presence of trauma, burns, or sepsis.

47. The treatment of choice for a duodenal ulcer is what procedure?
    a. Billroth II
    b. Billroth I
    c. Laparoscopic Nissen fundoplication
    d. Total gastrectomy

Answer: a. A Billroth II involves removal of the distal two thirds of the stomach with anastomosis to the jejunum. A Billroth I involves anastomosis to the duodenum, which doesn't treat the duodenal ulcer. A laparoscopic Nissen fundoplication is a treatment for GERD and a total gastrectomy is not indicated for a duodenal ulcer.

48. Complications of a duodenal ulcer is what?
    a. Zollinger-Ellison syndrome
    b. Pancreatic disease
    c. Chronic renal failure
    d. Hemorrhage

Answer: d. Hemorrhage is more common in a duodenal ulcer. Zollinger-Ellison syndrome, pancreatic disease and chronic renal failure are all precursors to duodenal ulcer.

49. The most lethal complication of a duodenal ulcer is what?
    a. Hemorrhage
    b. Perforation
    c. Gastric outlet obstruction
    d. H. pylori infection

Answer: b. Perforation is the most dangerous complication of a duodenal ulcer because it often leaks through the pancreas and leads to sepsis.

50. The main test to diagnose a duodenal ulcer is what test?
    a. Fiberoptic endoscopy with biopsy and detection of H. pylori
    b. H. pylori antibody titer
    c. Nissen fundoplication
    d. Upper GI Barium Swallow

Answer: a. The main test for a duodenal ulcer is a fiberoptic endoscopy with biopsy to detect H. pylori. An antibody titer for H. pylori does not identify an active disease state. A Nissen fundoplication is a treatment for GERD and an upper GI barium swallow is less effective when it comes to diagnosing a duodenal ulcer.

51. Nursing interventions for a duodenal ulcer include the following. Select all that apply.
    a. Aspirin for pain.
    b. NPO and NG to low intermittent suction
    c. Proton pump inhibitors
    d. Provide anticholinergics
    e. Feed small bland meals
    f. Liquid diet only

Answer: b. c. d. The nursing management of duodenal ulcers include NPO status with NG to low intermittent suction, anticholinergics, antacids, H2 blockers, proton pump inhibitors, and sedatives as ordered. Aspirin is contraindicated and there should be nothing by mouth.

52. Treatment of upper GI hemorrhage due to duodenal ulcer includes the following. Select all that apply.
    a. Provide a liquid diet only.
    b. NPO
    c. Eat soft, bland foods
    d. NG tube to decompress the stomach.
    e. Ice water lavage
    f. IV fluid and blood replacement

Answer: b. d. e. f. For a hemorrhage from a duodenal ulcer, you need to keep the client NPO, have an NG tube to decompress the stomach, provide ice water lavages and replace both IV fluids and blood.

53. The client has been diagnosed with acute appendicitis. What does the nurse tell the client in the way of education?
   a. The peak age of appendicitis is 65 years of age.
   b. It can be caused by a fecalith.
   c. It causes left lower quadrant abdominal pain.
   d. A major complication is hemorrhage.

Answer: b. The peak age of appendicitis is 11-30 years of age. It can be caused by a fecalith, tumor, foreign body or intramural thickening of the appendix. It causes right lower quadrant abdominal pain. The major complication is perforation.

54. A common complication of a Billroth II procedure is what?
   a. Pyloric stenosis
   b. Dumping syndrome
   c. Postoperative hemorrhage
   d. Peritonitis

Answer: b. A common complication of a Billroth II procedure is dumping syndrome. Postoperative hemorrhage and peritonitis are uncommon complications and the pylorus is removed as part of the procedure.

55. A client has dumping syndrome. What are common symptoms of dumping syndrome? Select all that apply.
    a. Diarrhea
    b. Vomiting
    c. Borborygmi
    d. Sweating
    e. Palpitations
    f. Lower abdominal pain

Answer: c. d. e. Common symptoms of dumping syndrome are abdominal cramps, urge to defecate, borborygmi, generalized weakness, sweating, palpitations, and dizziness within 30 minutes of meals.

56. The nurse is giving instructions to a client with dumping syndrome. What does the nurse recommend?
    a. Eat a large high protein diet
    b. Eat a small high carbohydrate diet rich in refined sugar
    c. Eat a small low carbohydrate diet with moderate fat and protein
    d. Drink clear liquids only

Answer: c. Eat a small low carbohydrate diet with moderate fat and protein for dumping syndrome. High proteins and fats can contribute to dumping syndrome and large meals can contribute to dumping syndrome. Clear liquids only is not necessary.

57. The client has postprandial hypoglycemia. As a nurse you tell the patient this:
    a. It results from eating too much complex carbohydrates.
    b. It is the result of eating too much concentrated simple carbohydrate.
    c. It is the result of insulin resistance.
    d. It is caused by eating too much protein in the diet.

Answer: b. Postprandial hypoglycemia is the result of eating too much concentrated simple carbohydrates.

58. The client has been diagnosed with bile reflux gastritis. What is a common treatment of the disorder?
    a. Antibiotics for H. pylori
    b. H2 blockers
    c. Questran before or with meals
    d. Low fat diet

Answer: c. One of the treatments o bile reflux gastritis is to give Questran in order to bind the bile acids and decrease the amount of irritant.

59. The client has been diagnosed with inflammatory bowel syndrome. What are some possible diagnoses? Select all that apply.
    a. Irritable bowel syndrome
    b. Chronic appendicitis
    c. Crohn's disease
    d. Acute colitis
    e. Ulcerative colitis
    f. H. pylori disease

Answer: c. e. The two types of inflammatory bowel syndrome are Crohn's disease and ulcerative colitis.

60. A client with an inflammatory disease wants to know the difference between Crohn's disease and ulcerative colitis. What does the nurse say?
    a. Crohn's disease is an autoimmune disease and ulcerative colitis is not.
    b. Crohn's disease can affect any part of the GI tract and ulcerative colitis affects just the colon.
    c. The onset of age of Crohn's disease is much older than that of those with ulcerative colitis.
    d. Crohn's disease presents with diarrhea, while ulcerative colitis presents with constipation.

Answer: b. Crohn's disease can affect any part of the GI tract, while ulcerative colitis affects just the colon.

61. The client with Crohn's disease wonders what complications can be expected. What does the nurse say? Select all that apply.
    a. Constipation
    b. Gastrointestinal stricture
    c. Weight gain
    d. Fat malabsorption
    e. Gluten intolerance
    f. Heartburn

Answer: b. d. e. Common complications of Crohn's disease are strictures, obstruction, fistulas, fat malabsorption, and gluten intolerance.

62. A diet for a client with Crohn's disease is what?
    a. High in protein and calories
    b. High in roughage
    c. High in fat
    d. High in milk

Answer: a. A diet or a person with Crohn's disease is one that is high in protein and calories, low in roughage, low in fat, low in residue, and milk-free.

63. Medical treatment for Crohn's disease includes:
    a. H2 blockers
    b. Protein pump inhibitors
    c. Azulfidine
    d. Laxatives

Answer: c. The major treatments for Crohn's disease include Azulfidine and corticosteroids. They generally do not need H2 blockers, proton pump inhibitors, or laxatives.

64. Chemical causes of peritonitis include what?
    a. Ruptured appendix
    b. Pancreatitis
    c. Perforated peptic ulcer
    d. Peritoneal dialysis

Answer: c. A perforated peptic ulcer or a ruptured ectopic pregnancy can cause a chemical peritonitis. Bacterial causes of peritonitis include a ruptured appendicitis, pancreatitis, GI obstruction, gunshot wound and peritoneal dialysis.

65. A client has acute peritonitis. What does the nurse say that complications of this condition are? Select all that apply.
    a. H. pylori infection
    b. Hypovolemic shock
    c. Constipation
    d. Septicemia
    e. Paralytic ileus
    f. Gallbladder dysfunction

Answer: b. d. e. Complications of acute peritonitis include hypovolemic shock, septicemia, paralytic ileus, intra-abdominal abscess, and organ failure.

66. A client has peritonitis. What are some nursing interventions that can be done? Select all that apply.
    a. Give oral ibuprofen or Tylenol
    b. NPO with NG suction
    c. Have the client lie on left side
    d. Give antibiotics as ordered
    e. Give IV fluids and electrolytes
    f. Give anti-emetics

Answer: b. d. e. A client with peritonitis should be placed on NPO status with NG suction. Antibiotics are given as ordered and the client should receive IV fluids and electrolytes. No oral intake is allowed so anti-emetics are not necessary. The client can be supine.

67. A client in the clinic is diagnosed with gastroenteritis. What do you tell the client about the condition?
    a. Antibiotics are usually recommended.
    b. It is caused by a virus.
    c. It is generally self-limited.
    d. It is usually treated with antacids.

Answer: c. Gastroenteritis is generally self-limited. It can be viral, bacterial or fungal. It generally does not require antibiotics. It is generally not treated with antacids.

68. A client has been diagnosed with ulcerative colitis. What do you tell the client as part of education?
    a. Any part of the GI tract can be affected.
    b. The most common age at onset is 30-40.
    c. It has a discontinuous disease process.
    d. A complication is toxic megacolon.

Answer: d. A complication of ulcerative colitis. It only affects the large colon and it affects the colon continuously. The peak age is 15 to 25 years of age. A complication is toxic megacolon.

69. A client with ulcerative colitis wonders about complications. What does the nurse tell the client? Select all that apply.
    a. Constipation
    b. H. pylori infection
    c. Hemorrhage
    d. Strictures
    e. Perforation
    f. Toxic megacolon

Answer: c. d. e. f. Complications include hemorrhage, strictures, perforation, toxic megacolon, and acute colitis.

70. A client has been diagnosed with diverticulosis. What does the nurse tell the client in terms of education?
    a. It is usually asymptomatic.
    b. It involves inflammation in the colon.
    c. The treatment is antibiotics.
    d. It is common in young adults.

Answer: a. Diverticulitis is usually asymptomatic. There is no inflammation of the colon and no antibiotics are required. It is more common in older adults.

71. A client has diverticulosis. What does the nurse tell the client about complications of this disorder?
    a. There are generally no complications of this disorder.
    b. Constipation can be a complication of this disorder.
    c. Diverticulitis can be a complication of this disorder.
    d. Diarrhea can be a complication of this disorder.

Answer: c. Diverticulitis is the main complication of diverticulitis.

72. A client has been diagnosed with diverticulitis. What can you tell the client about possible complications? Select all that apply.
    a. Diverticulosis is a complication.
    b. Peritonitis is a complication.
    c. Constipation is a complication.
    d. Bowel obstruction is a complication.
    e. Hemorrhage is a complication.
    f. Rectal prolapse is a complication.

Answer: b. d. e. Complications of diverticulitis include peritonitis, bowel obstruction and hemorrhage. Diverticulosis and constipation are causes of diverticulitis. Rectal prolapse is not a complication of diverticulitis.

73. The nurse is assessing the client for possible diverticulitis. What does the nurse look for? Select all that apply.
    a. Right lower quadrant abdominal pain.
    b. Fever and chills
    c. Nausea and vomiting
    d. Constipation
    e. Leukocytosis
    f. Diarrhea

Answer: b. c. e. In looking for diverticulitis, the nurse looks for left lower quadrant abdominal pain, nausea and vomiting, fever and chills, and leukocytosis. Constipation and diarrhea are generally non-specific findings.

74. The client has acute diverticulitis. What does the nurse say about the risks of doing a colonoscopy for the diagnosis of the disease?
    a. It is less risky than a barium enema.
    b. It can cause perforation and peritonitis.
    c. There are no risks in doing the colonoscopy.
    d. It can cause diverticulosis to become diverticulitis.

Answer: b. The colonoscopy is riskier than a barium enema in acute diverticulitis because it can result in bowel perforation and peritonitis. It cannot cause diverticulosis to become diverticulitis.

75. The client has diverticulitis. What nursing interventions do you perform? Select all that apply.
    a. Instruct the client in selecting low fiber foods.
    b. Tell the client to drink more fluids.
    c. Tell the client to take anti-diarrheals.
    d. Administer bulk laxatives.
    e. Tell the client to gain some weight.
    f. Provide antibiotics as ordered.

Answer: b. d. f. The nurse should help the client select high fiber foods, drink more fluids, take bulk laxatives and anticholinergics, and lose weight, which decreases intra-abdominal pressure. The nurse should also provide antibiotics as ordered.

76. The client is having a total colectomy with ileal reservoir. How do you educate the client about the procedure?
    a. Tell them it is actually two procedures done 8-12 weeks apart.
    b. Tell them it involves removal of part of the colon.
    c. The person ends up with a reanastomosis in the end.
    d. The goal is to increase the number of stools daily.

Answer: a. The procedure is actually two procedures done 8-12 weeks apart. The first part is removal of the entire colon and rectal mucosectomy, construction of ileal reservoir, and anastomosis with temporary ileostomy. The second procedure involves closure of the ileostomy when the capacity of the reservoir is increased. The goal is to decrease the number of stools daily.

77. The client presents with a strangulated hernia. What does the nurse tell the client about this condition?
    a. It is generally not painful.
    b. It occurs when the hernia is fully reducible into the abdominal cavity.
    c. It can lead to diarrhea.
    d. It happens when the intestinal flow and blood supply is obstructed.

Answer: d. A strangulated hernia involves obstruction of the blood flow and intestinal flow of a portion of the intestines. It is generally painful. It does not generally lead to diarrhea.

78. The diagnosis of a strangulated abdominal hernia involves what?
   a. A barium enema
   b. A colonoscopy
   c. An abdominal x-ray
   d. An upper GI endoscopy

Answer: c. An abdominal x-ray will reveal an obstruction in the intestinal tract. The other choices are not indicated in the diagnosis of a strangulated abdominal hernia.

79. A client has just had repair of an inguinal hernia. What does the nurse instruct the client to do? Select all that apply.
   a. No lifting greater than 50 pounds for 2 weeks.
   b. Put an ice bag onto the scrotal area after surgery.
   c. Coughing is discouraged.
   d. The stitches are always dissolvable and nothing more needs to be done.
   e. Return to the hospital if excessive urination occurs.
   f. Sneeze with the mouth opened.

Answer: b. c. f. The client should not lift anything heavy for 6-8 weeks. An ice bag should be put on the scrotal area to decrease swelling. Coughing is discouraged and the client should sneeze with the mouth open. There can be a problem with decreased urination so a catheter may have to be placed. Sutures may or may not be dissolvable.

80. A client has external hemorrhoids. What does the nurse tell the client about the causes of the condition? Select all that apply.
    a. Loose stools
    b. Prolonged standing or sitting
    c. Diverticulosis
    d. Pregnancy
    e. Lean body mass
    f. Portal hypertension

Answer: b. d. f. Common causes of hemorrhoids include straining at stool, prolonged sitting or standing, pregnancy, obesity, and portal hypertension.

81. A child is scheduled for hernia repair. What type of hernia is the child likely to have?
    a. Inguinal hernia
    b. Femoral hernia
    c. Ventral hernia
    d. Umbilical hernia

Answer: d. Children are more likely to suffer from umbilical hernias in which the umbilical area fails to close after birth.

82. The client has a type of hepatitis gotten from exposure to contaminated food. What type of hepatitis does this client likely have?
    a. Hepatitis A
    b. Hepatitis B
    c. Hepatitis C
    d. Hepatitis D

Answer: a. Of the types of hepatitis, only hepatitis A is the result of eating food contaminated with the virus.

83. A client has been diagnosed with hemorrhoids. What are some nursing interventions the nurse can do? Select all that apply.
    a. Tell the client to eat a low fiber diet.
    b. Restrict fluids.
    c. Use ointments for pain such as Nupercainal.
    d. Apply ice packs alternating with warm packs.
    e. Give analgesics after defecation.
    f. Offer warm sitz baths

Answer: c. d. f. The nurse should tell the client to eat a high fiber diet, push fluids, use ointments such as Nupercainal, apply ice packs alternating with warm packs, give analgesics before defecation and offer warm sitz baths.

84. The client has been diagnosed with hepatitis B. How do you educate the client?
    a. The Incubation period is 2-4 weeks.
    b. The transmission is through the fecal-oral route.
    c. It is transmitted through accidental needle sticks.
    d. The condition resolves in about ten weeks.

Answer: c. This type of hepatitis can be transmitted by accidental needle sticks, blood transfusions, organ transplantation or sexual activity. The incubation time is 7-24 weeks. Not everyone recovers from the disorder and there are chronic carriers.

85. What is a serious complication of hepatitis C?
    a. Liver cirrhosis
    b. Liver cancer
    c. Hemodialysis
    d. Liver flukes

Answer: c. A serious complication of hepatitis C is liver cancer. Hemodialysis, tattooing, blood transfusions and sexual activity with a contaminated partner are causes of hepatitis C.

86. A client from a developing country has been diagnosed with hepatitis E. What do you tell the client as a way of education?
    a. It is spread by blood transfusions and sex with a contaminated partner.
    b. It is common in the US.
    c. It is spread by contaminated drinking water.
    d. It has a 10-12 week incubation stage.

Answer: c. It is spread by contaminated drinking water, usually from developing countries. It is uncommon in the US and has an incubation time of 2-8 weeks.

87. A client has hepatitis A. What do you tell the client when asked about ways to prevent the disease?
    a. Use condoms when having sex.
    b. Use scrupulous handwashing when dealing with food.
    c. Do not get a blood transfusion.
    d. Immune globulin provides permanent prevention.

Answer: b. To protect against hepatitis A, the client must use scrupulous hand washing when dealing with food. Immune globulin provides temporary protection against the disease. Only a hepatitis A vaccination will provide permanent protection against the disease.

88. The client has just been diagnosed with cirrhosis of the liver due to alcoholism. What do you tell the client in the way of education?
    a. It is an acute inflammation of the liver that can last up to 6 months.
    b. It is most common in women around age 30.
    c. It has a high mortality rate.
    d. The most common cause is hepatitis B

Answer: c. Cirrhosis is a chronic condition of the liver with the most likely cause being alcoholism. It occurs mostly in men around 50 years of age. It has a high mortality rate.

89. The client has hepatitis and wonders about the disease. What do you tell the client about the phases of hepatitis?
    a. The preicteric phase occurs in the absence of jaundice.
    b. The icteric phase involves severe left upper quadrant abdominal pain.
    c. The posticteric phase lasts about a month.
    d. The preclimactic phase involves fever, chills, and malaise.

Answer: a. The preicteric phase involves an absence of jaundice. The icteric phase involves jaundice and the reduction of fever. The posticteric phase lasts 2-4 months. There is no preclimactic phase.

90. The client has hepatitis. What are some nursing interventions the nurse can do? Select all that apply.
    a. Encourage activity
    b. Engage in meticulous oral care.
    c. Encourage a weight loss diet.
    d. Give anti-emetics for nausea.
    e. Give laxatives for constipation.
    f. Weigh the client daily

Answer: b. d. f. The client should have bedrest and meticulous oral care. Encourage a high calorie diet and give anti-emetics for nausea. The client should be weighed daily.

91. The patient has acute pancreatitis. What does the nurse say about the causes of pancreatitis?
    a. It can be caused by gallbladder disease.
    b. It can be caused by hepatitis.
    c. It can be caused by peptic acid disease.
    d. It can be caused by hyperlipidemia.
    e. It can be caused by alcoholism.
    f. It can be caused by hypoparathyroid conditions.

Answer: a. d. e. Pancreatitis can be caused by biliary tract disease, alcoholism, surgical trauma, penetrating duodenal ulcer, hyperparathyroidism, hyperlipidemia, renal failure, certain drugs such as thiazide diuretics, oral contraceptives, corticosteroids, NSAIDs, and sulfonamides and following endoscopic retrograde cholangiopancreatography (ERCP).

92. A common complication of pancreatitis includes the following:
    a. Sepsis
    b. Pancreatic pseudocyst
    c. Dehydration
    d. Diarrhea

Answer: b. The two most common complications of pancreatitis are pancreatic pseudocyst and abscess formation. It does not cause sepsis, dehydration or diarrhea, as a rule.

93. The client has severe, left upper quadrant pain radiating to the back that is made worse by eating and is not relieved by vomiting. The client wants to flex the spine in order to relieve the pain and shows evidence of flushing, cyanosis, dyspnea, and nausea/vomiting. What does the client likely have?
    a. Peptic acid disease
    b. GERD
    c. Acute cholecystitis
    d. Acute pancreatitis

Answer: d. The client with this set of signs and symptoms likely has acute pancreatitis. Evaluation will show elevated WBCs, elevated amylase, and elevated lipase.

94. The client is complaining of a heavy, gnawing paint in the left upper quadrant of the abdomen, weight loss, malabsorption, steatorrhea, mild jaundice and diabetes. What does the client likely have?
    a. Peptic ulcer disease
    b. Acute cholecystitis
    c. Chronic pancreatitis
    d. GERD

Answer: c. The symptoms and signs are most consistent with chronic pancreatitis. A serum amylase and serum lipase will be elevated.

95. The client has cirrhosis. What do you tell the client about the possible causes and types of cirrhosis? Select all that apply.
    a. Cirrhosis can be caused by a complication of viral, autoimmune or toxic hepatitis.
    b. Cirrhosis can be caused by peptic acid disease.
    c. Cirrhosis can be caused by GERD.
    d. Cirrhosis can be caused by biliary obstruction and infection
    e. Cirrhosis can be caused by right-sided heart failure.
    f. Cirrhosis can be caused by acute pancreatitis.

Answer: a. d. e. Cirrhosis can be caused by hepatitis that causes scar tissue in the liver, biliary obstruction and infection, and by right-sided heart failure.

96. Complications of liver cirrhosis include the following? Select all that apply.
    a. Acute peptic ulcer
    b. Acute pancreatitis
    c. Hepatic encephalopathy
    d. Portal hypertension with ascites
    e. Coma
    f. Gallbladder disease

Answer: c. d. e. Complications of cirrhosis of the liver include portal hypertension, jaundice, esophageal varices, peripheral edema, ascites, renal failure, hepatic encephalopathy, and coma.

97. A client with liver cirrhosis has fector hepaticus. What do you tell the client that this is?
    a. The type of coma associated with increased ammonia levels.
    b. Steatorrhea from cirrhosis
    c. A musty, sweet breath odor
    d. Right upper quadrant abdominal fullness.

Answer: c. Tell the client that fector hepaticus is a musty, sweet odor to the breath.

98. Nursing interventions for patients with liver cirrhosis include the following. Select all that apply.
    a. Give Questran for itching
    b. Increase activity
    c. Reduce liquid intake.
    d. Offer between meal snacks
    e. Meticulous skin care
    f. Eat a high fat diet

Answer: a. d. e. Nursing interventions for patients with liver cirrhosis include giving Questran for itching, bed rest, monitor intake and output, monitor daily weights, offer between meal snacks and meticulous skin care.

99. The client has been diagnosed with acute cholecystitis. What do you tell the client about complications of the disease? Select all that apply.
    a. Acute cholangitis
    b. Obesity
    c. Pancreatitis
    d. Biliary cirrhosis
    e. Duodenal ulcer
    f. Peptic ulcer

Answer: a. c. d. Acute cholecystitis has the following complications: cholangitis, pancreatitis, biliary cirrhosis, carcinoma, and peritonitis.

100.   Diagnostic tests for acute cholelithiasis include:
a. MRI of the abdomen
b. CT scan of the abdomen
c. Ultrasound of the gallbladder
d. Liver function tests
e. Oral cholecystogram
f. Upper GI endoscopy

Answer: c. d. e. Tests for acute cholelithiasis include ultrasonography, oral cholecystogram, IV cholangiogram, percutaneous transhepatic cholangiography, liver function tests, white blood cell count, and serum enzymes. CT and MRI are not necessary tests and an upper GI endoscopy will not help.

101. The client has acute pancreatitis. What nursing interventions do you do? Select all that apply.
a. Help them assume the pain relief positions.
b. NPO and jejunostomy tube
c. Lactated Ringers by IV
d. Insulin for low blood sugar
e. Encourage activity to decrease pain
f. Encourage high fat meals

Answer: a. b. c. The nurse should help the client assume the pain relief positions, put the client on NPO with a jejunostomy tube, give Lactated Ringers by IV, give insulin for high blood sugar, rest and give them small high carb and high protein/low fat meals.

102. For a client with chronic pancreatitis, what do you give the patient for treatment as ordered?
   a. Give pancreatin and pancrelipase
   b. Give metformin for blood sugars
   c. Give Demerol for pain
   d. Give thiazide diuretics for edema

Answer: a. The client should receive pancreatin and pancrelipase to replace pancreatic enzymes. They should receive insulin and not metformin for blood sugars. Demerol is contraindicated because of toxicity and the client with chronic pancreatitis would receive Lasix for edema.

103. A client has cholelithiasis. What do you tell the client in the way of education?
   a. There is no way to dissolve the stones.
   b. An extracorporeal shock-wave lithotripsy can be used to dissolve stones.
   c. Pancreatin is necessary for replacing pancreatic enzymes.
   d. You will have to take metformin for high blood sugar.

Answer: b. Tell the client that an extracorporeal shock-wave lithotripsy can be used to dissolve stones. Pancreatic is not indicated and, if there is pancreatitis, insulin is recommended.

104. The nurse is evaluating the abdomen. What subjective assessment should be included?
   a. Generalized abdominal rash
   b. Rebound tenderness
   c. Diarrhea
   d. Hematuria

Answer: b. Of the above findings, only rebound tenderness is considered subjective.

105. A client has just had an upper GI endoscopy. What should the nurse do as part of nursing interventions?
   a. Help the client maintain the right-side lying position.
   b. Give the client a fatty test meal.
   c. Keep the client NPO until the gag reflex returns.
   d. Give the client a bulk-forming laxative.

Answer: c. In caring for the client after an upper GI endoscopy, you must help them maintain a left-side lying position and should keep them NPO until the gag reflex returns.

CONCLUSION

Congrats! You did it! Remember, practice makes perfect so you may want to repeat these questions to make you feel more confident for the big exam day.

If you enjoyed this book, would you be kind enough to leave a review on Amazon? Your review can help others to see what kinds of helpful resources are out there!

Thank you and good luck on your medical endeavors! I'll talk to you soon and see you in the next book!

- Chase Hassen

Nurse Superhero

Made in the USA
Las Vegas, NV
04 August 2022